I0702176

BRONCHIECTASIS

Expert Guide to bronchiectasis Causes, Symptoms, Treatment, and Achieving Complete Wellness

DR. DASHIELL DANIEL

Copyright © DR. DASHIELL DANIEL 2023

All rights reserved.

No part of this publication may be reproduced, distributed, or transmitted in any form or by any means, including photocopying, recording, or other electronic or mechanical methods, without the prior written permission of the publisher, except in the case of brief quotations embodied in critical reviews and certain other non-commercial uses permitted by copyright law.

Disclaimer

This book, is intended to provide information and guidance on the subject matter and is not a substitute for professional medical advice, diagnosis, or treatment.

The author, is not a medical professional, and the content presented here is based on research, general knowledge, and expert guidance available at the time of writing.

The information in this book is provided with the understanding that the author and the publisher are not engaged in rendering medical, legal, or other professional services.

Any reliance on the information contained in this book is at the reader's own risk.

While every effort has been made to ensure the accuracy and completeness of the information presented, medical knowledge is constantly evolving, and new research may supersede the content in this book. The author and the publisher make no representations or warranties of any kind, express or implied, about the completeness, accuracy, reliability, suitability, or availability concerning the information, products, services, or related graphics contained in this book.

This book may contain references or mentions of individuals, products, websites, organizations, or other names for informational purposes only.

The author does not own or endorse any such entities mentioned in the book. Any resemblance to actual persons, living or dead, or actual events is purely coincidental.

Readers are encouraged to consult with qualified healthcare professionals for medical advice, diagnosis, and treatment tailored to their specific circumstances.

The author and the publisher disclaim any liability for any loss or risk, personal or otherwise, arising directly or indirectly from the use of the information presented in this book.

By reading this book, the reader acknowledges and agrees to the terms of this disclaimer.

"Bronchiectasis" is a book that offers a thorough examination of a respiratory disease that has significant consequences for patients and medical personnel. The work starts with a perceptive Introduction that explores the meaning and background of bronchiectasis, laying the foundation for a full comprehension of its importance. The significance of understanding bronchiectasis within the larger medical context is emphasized in this first chapter.

Chapter 1 of the book provides a comprehensive analysis of the anatomy and physiology of the respiratory system, providing a detailed synopsis of the complex structures and processes that support respiratory health. The function of bronchi is covered in detail, laying the groundwork for the next chapters. The reader's comprehension is furthered by Chapter 2, which clarifies the intricacies of bronchiectasis, including its diagnosis, categorization, causes, and risk factors. Notably, the investigation of both infectious and non-infectious origins highlights the complex character of this illness, and a thorough understanding of its pathophysiology improves clinical judgment.

In Chapter 3, the signs and symptoms of bronchiectasis are discussed, along with an explanation of the clinical presentations that help with diagnosis. The next chapter, Diagnosis, describes in detail the diagnostic modalities—such as imaging scans, microbiological testing, and clinical evaluation—that are necessary to accurately and promptly diagnose bronchiectasis.

Chapter 5, which delves deeply into the Treatment and Management of bronchiectasis, is the central section of the book. Surgical alternatives, lifestyle changes, pharmaceutical therapies, and chest physical therapy are all covered in great depth, giving researchers and physicians a wealth of information to help them make well-informed decisions.

As it acknowledges the comprehensive requirements of those impacted by bronchiectasis, Chapter 6 takes a compassionate turn, delving into the human side of the illness in "Living with Bronchiectasis." Coping methods, supportive care, and patient education are covered.

Finally, Chapter 7 of the book explores how bronchiectasis research is developing.

Future prospects, cutting-edge treatments, and current research trends are explored to provide an early look at the developments that might influence bronchiectasis care in the years to come.

"Bronchiectasis" is essentially a valuable resource that connects the gaps between professional knowledge, patient experience, and potential future developments. This scientific effort fosters a deeper knowledge of bronchiectasis and paves the road for better care and results. It is a lighthouse for scholars, healthcare professionals, and people living with the condition.

Overview

A chronic respiratory disease called bronchiectasis is characterized by irreversible bronchial and bronchiole dilatation and destruction, which can result in recurring and persistent infections.

Mucus and bacteria build up in the afflicted airways as a result of this illness, which sets off a vicious cycle of inflammation and more structural damage. The quality of life can be significantly impacted by bronchiectasis, which frequently manifests as symptoms including a persistent cough, copious sputum production, and recurring respiratory infections. Healthcare providers must be well-versed in the complexities of bronchiectasis to diagnose patients accurately, treat them effectively, and help them achieve better results.

What Bronchiectasis Means

A chronic respiratory condition known as bronchiectasis is characterized by aberrant, persistent bronchial and bronchiole dilatation, poor mucus clearance, and recurrent bacterial infections. The breakdown of the airway walls' musculoskeletal and elastic components causes this dilatation and a lack of structural integrity. Because the injured bronchi are unable to remove mucus efficiently, it builds up and creates the perfect conditions for the development of germs. Based on the cause of the illness, bronchiectasis may be categorized into three main types: idiopathic bronchiectasis, post-infectious bronchiectasis, and bronchiectasis linked with cystic fibrosis. Comprehending the particular etiology is essential for customizing therapeutic strategies and tackling the fundamental reasons.

An Overview Of The Past

The historical background of bronchiectasis shows how our knowledge of the ailment has evolved throughout time. At first, the cause of bronchiectasis was unknown and it was frequently thought to be a side effect of other respiratory illnesses. As medical knowledge grew, especially in the 19th and 20th centuries, bronchiectasis was identified by specialists as a separate condition. The development of diagnostic techniques like bronchoscopy and chest imaging allowed for a more thorough examination of the anatomical alterations in the airways linked to bronchiectasis. This historical voyage highlights the value of ongoing investigation and advancement in medicine in deciphering the intricacies of bronchiectasis, culminating in enhanced diagnostic methods and treatment strategies.

The Value Of Knowing About Bronchiectasis

Given the substantial clinical consequences of bronchiectasis, understanding of the condition is essential. First and foremost, a precise diagnosis is essential to distinguish bronchiectasis from other respiratory disorders that present with comparable symptoms, such as asthma or chronic obstructive pulmonary disease (COPD).

A misdiagnosis may lead to improper management techniques and a postponed start of targeted therapy. Moreover, customizing treatment strategies requires an understanding of the many etiological elements that contribute to bronchiectasis. For example, successful management of bronchiectasis requires addressing the underlying cause, such as treating repeated infections or controlling cystic fibrosis.

Additionally, creating preventative measures requires a thorough understanding of bronchiectasis. Identifying risk factors and taking steps to reduce them can assist those who are prone to bronchiectasis to prevent the disease from progressing. This is especially important when bronchiectasis is brought on by repeated respiratory infections or exposure to the environment. Campaigns for education and public health can be extremely effective in increasing public knowledge of bronchiectasis, its risk factors, and the value of early intervention.

Furthermore, increasing treatment choices for bronchiectasis depends on further study. It is necessary to keep focusing on developing new therapeutic approaches, examining the part inflammation plays in the development of disease, and finding biomarkers for early detection.

As our knowledge of bronchiectasis advances, so do the prospects for creating more specialized and potent therapies, which will eventually enhance the prognosis and standard of living for those who suffer from this persistent respiratory ailment.

bronchiectasis is a complicated respiratory condition with many facets that affect a person's life in many ways. By gaining a thorough comprehension of the definition, historical background, and clinical significance of bronchiectasis, medical practitioners may effectively manage the difficulties presented by the condition, resulting in better patient outcomes, more accurate diagnoses, and customized treatment plans.

CHAPTER ONE
ANATOMY AND PHYSIOLOGY OF THE RESPIRATORY SYSTEM

The intricate network of tissues and organs that make up the respiratory system is essential for the exchange of gases between the body and its surroundings. It is made up of the lower and upper respiratory tracts, each of which has unique physical features and purposes. The throat, larynx, and nasal passages are all part of the upper respiratory system; the trachea, bronchi, bronchioles, and lungs are all part of the lower respiratory tract. Together, these elements enable the body's metabolic functions by facilitating the absorption of oxygen and the expulsion of carbon dioxide.

The Lungs' Structure And Function

The respiratory system's vital organs, the lungs, are crucial to gas exchange. The lungs are two spongy organs that are confined to the thoracic cavity. The lungs, which are made up of lobes, bronchi, bronchioles, and alveoli, are very well-designed to maximize breathing efficiency.

After emerging from the trachea, the bronchi further split into smaller bronchioles, which lead to clusters of air sacs called alveoli. To facilitate the exchange of oxygen and carbon dioxide during respiration, the alveoli are encircled by a vast network of capillaries and bordered by a thin layer of epithelial cells. The lungs' ability to produce surfactants and their elastic nature both aid in effective ventilation and the prevention of alveolar collapse.

The Bronchi's Function In The Respiratory System

The trachea and the lungs are connected by the bronchi, which are important airways in the respiratory system. These tube structures split, creating bronchioles that get smaller and smaller in diameter. Mucus-producing goblet cells and ciliated epithelial cells are features of the bronchi that together support the mucociliary clearance process. By capturing and eliminating inhaled particles and germs, this process helps stop them from penetrating deeper lung tissues. The bronchi are also essential for controlling airflow and delivering air uniformly throughout the lungs' different regions.

Bronchiectasis

A chronic respiratory disease called bronchiectasis is characterized by irreversible bronchial and bronchiole dilatation and destruction. Recurrent lung infections, persistent inflammation, or other underlying lung illnesses are frequently the cause of this pathology. The bronchial wall becomes compromised due to ongoing inflammation and structural damage, which widens the airways and causes an excess of mucus to build up.

As a result, mucus clearance is hampered, which worsens respiratory function and increases the risk of recurring infections.

The delicate balance needed for effective breathing processes is impacted by the disruption of the normal architecture of the bronchi in bronchiectasis.

Chronic dilatation of the airways produces pockets where mucus collects, which is the perfect setting for the development of germs. This feeds back into a vicious cycle of infection, inflammation, and structural damage, which makes bronchiectasis more progressive.

Respiratory symptoms include persistent cough, sputum production, and recurring respiratory infections are caused by the lungs' inability to efficiently filter, humidify, and oxygenate incoming air due to damaged bronchi and reduced mucociliary clearance.

Possible Effects On The Respiratory System

Significant effects on the respiratory system's morphology and physiology result from bronchiectasis.

Chronic bronchial dilatation modifies the regular dynamics of airflow, making it more difficult for air to be distributed to the different parts of the lungs effectively. The impaired mucociliary clearance reduces the effectiveness of the system's filtering and removal of airborne particles and microorganisms. Moreover, the anatomical harm to the bronchi upsets the delicate equilibrium between airway resistance and patency, which increases airflow restriction and respiratory discomfort.

Bronchiectasis affects more than only the anatomical modifications to the respiratory system. This condition's ongoing inflammation and infection can cause gradual lung damage that eventually compromises lung function as a whole. Hypoxemia and hypercapnia are caused by respiratory insufficiency, which is exacerbated by the poor gas exchange in injured bronchi and bronchioles. With time, this respiratory impairment may have systemic effects that impact bronchiectasis patients' cardiovascular health, ability to tolerate physical exertion, and general quality of life.

Methods For Diagnosing And Tracking

Effective care of bronchiectasis depends on a precise diagnosis and ongoing observation. High-resolution computed tomography (HRCT) scans are one type of diagnostic modality that may be used to identify bronchiectasis.

These scans give precise pictures of the bronchial architecture and can detect structural abnormalities and dilations. Tests for lung function called pulmonary function tests (PFTs) identify patterns of airflow restriction and impairment. Targeted therapy strategies can be guided by identifying the microbiological pathogens responsible for recurring infections using sputum culture and analysis.

Clinical examinations, lung function tests, and imaging investigations are required to track the development of bronchiectasis.

Regular evaluations assist medical practitioners in customizing treatment regimens to meet changing respiratory issues, maximize therapeutic interventions, and lessen condition-related consequences. For thorough management and better patient outcomes, multidisciplinary care involving pulmonologists, respiratory therapists, and infectious disease experts is essential.

Strategies For Treatment

The goals of bronchiectasis care are to reduce symptoms, avoid flare-ups, and enhance breathing capacity. Pharmacological therapies consist of antibiotics to treat bacterial infections, bronchodilators to improve airflow, and mucolytics to decrease mucus viscosity.

Programs for pulmonary rehabilitation include education, fitness training, and psychological support to improve patients' respiratory and general health. Mucus is mobilized and removed from the airways with the use of airway clearance procedures including positive expiratory pressure devices and chest physical therapy.

Immunization against respiratory pathogens is essential for avoiding infections that worsen bronchiectasis, especially pneumococcus and influenza. A thorough management strategy should also include lifestyle improvements, such as quitting smoking and altering the surroundings to limit exposure to respiratory irritants. Surgical treatments like lung transplantation or bronchial artery embolization may be taken into consideration in extreme situations.

A complicated interaction between anatomical and physiological alterations in the respiratory system results in bronchiectasis.

Gaining knowledge of the minute aspects of the anatomy and physiology of the respiratory system provides the groundwork for understanding the pathophysiology and clinical presentations of bronchiectasis. The aforementioned condition's chronic and progressive nature highlights the criticality of prompt diagnosis, thorough monitoring, and interdisciplinary care to maximize patient outcomes. Healthcare providers can customize therapies to improve quality of life, improve respiratory function, and lessen the long-term effects of bronchiectasis by addressing the structural and functional abnormalities this chronic respiratory disease causes.

CHAPTER TWO
A COMPREHENSIVE GLOBAL APPROACH

The chronic respiratory disease bronchiectasis is typified by the permanent enlargement and destruction of the bronchi, which are the airways that provide oxygen to the lungs.

The buildup of mucus and recurrent respiratory infections caused by this crippling illness cause the function of the lungs to gradually deteriorate.

An in-depth examination of the description, categorization, etiology, risk factors, and complex pathophysiological mechanisms behind the appearance of bronchiectasis is necessary for a thorough investigation of the condition.

Meaning And Categorization

The abnormal and persistent enlargement of the bronchi, or branching airways inside the lungs, is known as bronchiectasis.

This dilatation frequently happens as a result of persistent infection and inflammation, which damages the bronchial walls structurally.

The origin and anatomical distribution of the illness allows for its classification into many kinds. Varicose bronchiectasis is characterized by sporadic, bead-like bronchial dilatation, whereas cylindrical bronchiectasis causes consistent bronchial dilatation. Conversely, the hallmark of cystic bronchiectasis is localized airway dilatation that resembles a sac. Comprehending these classes is essential to customizing successful treatment plans.

Reasons And Danger Elements

A variety of infectious and non-infectious factors can contribute to the beginning of bronchiectasis, making it a complex disease. A variety of respiratory diseases, including pneumonia, TB, and fungal infections, fall under the category of infectious causes.

These illnesses have the potential to cause long-term inflammation and consequent damage to the bronchi. Autoimmune conditions like rheumatoid arthritis, which can induce immune-mediated damage to the airways, are examples of non-infectious causes.

Due to predisposing factors such as cystic fibrosis, bronchiectasis is also influenced by genetics. Exposure to harmful chemicals and other environmental variables increases the likelihood of acquiring this chronic respiratory disease.

The Pathogenesis Of Bronchiectasis

A complicated interaction between inflammatory processes compromised mucociliary clearance, and structural alterations to the airways underlies the pathogenesis of bronchiectasis.

Inflammatory mediators and enzymes are released during chronic inflammation, which is frequently brought on by recurring infections and deteriorates bronchial walls.

As a result, the airways' structural integrity and elastic recoil are lost.

The dilated bronchi's mucus buildup is made worse by the compromised mucociliary clearance, a process that typically aids in the removal of germs and mucus. Mucus stasis and chronic inflammation together provide an environment that is favorable to bacterial colonization, which feeds the cycle of recurring infections and exacerbations. This process eventually leads to the development of bronchiectasis, which is the clinical expression of irreparable bronchial injury.

a complete investigation of the diagnosis, categorization, etiology, and complex pathophysiological mechanisms behind the disease's course is necessary to comprehend bronchiectasis. This information is crucial for the creation of focused treatment strategies meant to manage and enhance the quality of life for those suffering from this persistent respiratory ailment.

CHAPTER THREE
INDICATIONS AND SYMPTOMS

A chronic respiratory disease called bronchiectasis is characterized by permanent bronchial and bronchiole dilatation and destruction, which impairs airway clearance and increases the risk of recurring infections.

Although the signs and symptoms of bronchiectasis might differ from person to person, they usually present as a persistent cough, copious amounts of sputum, recurrent respiratory infections, hemoptysis, and other related issues.

Prolonged Cough

A chronic and persistent cough is one of the main signs and symptoms of bronchiectasis. Sputum is frequently discharged along with this cough, indicating that it is productive. Mucus builds up in the dilated and damaged airways, causing the cough, which is the body's natural reaction to clean the airways.

The patient's quality of life may be greatly impacted by the chronic nature of the cough, which can cause weariness, sleep difficulties, and psychological discomfort.

To effectively treat bronchiectasis, the underlying reasons for the patient's chronic cough must be addressed, and measures to lessen its interference with daily living must be put in place.

A Surplus Of Sputum Production

Another defining symptom of bronchiectasis is the excessive production of sputum, which is caused by increased mucus production in the damaged airways and persistent inflammation.

The production of viscous, difficult-to-clear sputum frequently contributes to airway blockage.

This ongoing accumulation of mucus serves as a haven for germs, raising the risk of respiratory infections even more.

A multimodal strategy is necessary to manage high sputum production, including mucolytic medicines, airway clearing procedures, and treating underlying causes such as infection and chronic inflammation.

Recurrent Chest Infections

People with bronchiectasis are more likely to experience recurring respiratory infections because their damaged and dilated airways are more prone to bacterial colonization.

These infections can exacerbate symptoms and present as pneumonia or bronchitis.

Although frequent antibiotic courses could be required to treat these illnesses, the danger of antibiotic resistance emphasizes the significance of a focused and prudent strategy.

Vaccination against respiratory pathogens, preservation of lung function, and treatment of underlying conditions that contribute to the increased susceptibility to infections are long-term management methods.

Hemoptysis

One worrisome sign of bronchiectasis is hemoptysis, or coughing up blood from the respiratory tract. Blood in sputum can occur from the burst of damaged blood vessels within dilated airways. Hemostasis can range in severity from little streaks to larger volumes of blood, but it always has to be treated very away.

It is essential to determine the underlying cause of hemoptysis since it may be a sign of an infection, inflammation, or other issues. As part of treatment, the patient must be stabilized, the underlying cause must be addressed, and steps must be taken to stop the bleeding from continuing.

Additional Signs And Complications

In addition to the primary symptoms, bronchiectasis can result in several other symptoms and consequences.

Because of the increased energy expenditure brought on by persistent coughing and illness, fatigue and weight loss may result.

People with bronchiectasis may have reductions in their total functional ability and tolerance to exercise as the condition advances.

Furthermore, in extreme cases, complications including cor pulmonale and respiratory failure may occur, highlighting the necessity for comprehensive care techniques that address both the systemic and pulmonary elements of the disorder.

hemoptysis, recurrent respiratory infections, excessive sputum production, persistent cough, and a variety of related problems are the hallmarks of the complicated clinical picture of bronchiectasis. Developing successful therapy options that include both symptomatic relief and treating the underlying causes of the ailment requires an understanding of the complex nature of these indications and symptoms.

The goal of ongoing research and therapeutic developments is to enhance the quality of life and prognosis for people with bronchiectasis, underscoring the need for a multidisciplinary approach to these patients' treatment.

CHAPTER FOUR
DIAGNOSIS

Chronic bronchiectasis is a respiratory disease marked by irreversible bronchial and bronchiole dilatation, which causes inflammation of the airways and recurring infections. A multifaceted approach is used to diagnose bronchiectasis, including imaging examinations, lung function tests, microbiological testing, and clinical evaluation.

A crucial part of diagnosing bronchiectasis is clinical assessment. The foundation is the patient's history, which offers important information about the beginning, course, and development of symptoms. It is also essential to thoroughly investigate risk factors such as a family history of respiratory disorders, exposure to environmental toxins, and recurring respiratory infections. Sputum production, hemoptysis, persistent cough, and recurring chest infections are examples of suggestive symptoms that need to be properly brought up during the patient interview.

Another crucial element of the clinical evaluation for the diagnosis of bronchiectasis is the physical examination. Wheezing and harsh crackles may be audible during chest auscultation, and digital clubbing—a telltale symptom of long-term respiratory disorders—may be seen upon closer examination. It's important to take a close look at any respiratory distress symptoms including cyanosis. Clinicians can make a preliminary diagnosis and determine whether more diagnostic tests are necessary with the use of the patient history and physical examination results.

To determine the severity of bronchiectasis and to confirm the diagnosis, imaging investigations are necessary. While they might not be as sensitive as other imaging modalities, chest X-rays offer a baseline evaluation. Because high-resolution CT scans are better at seeing abnormalities in the airways, they are regarded as the gold standard for diagnosing bronchiectasis.

A thorough evaluation of bronchial dilatation, mucous plugging, and the presence of thickening of the bronchial wall is made possible by CT scans. The distinguishing characteristics of imaging aid in the differentiation of bronchiectasis from other respiratory disorders and direct the development of a suitable treatment strategy.

PFTs, or pulmonary function tests, are essential for assessing how bronchiectasis affects function. Measurements such as forced expiratory volume in one second (FEV1) and forced vital capacity (FVC) are used in spirometry to evaluate lung function. Reduction in FEV1 and restriction of airflow are frequent findings in bronchiectasis. Evaluation of lung volumes and diffusing capacity contributes to the understanding of the disease's severity and helps track the course of the illness over time.

For individuals with bronchiectasis, microbiological testing is essential in determining the microbial pathogens causing recurrent respiratory infections.

Antibiotic susceptibility of bacterial strains is ascertained and identified with the use of sputum culture and sensitivity testing. A typical symptom of bronchiectasis is chronic bacterial colonization, with prevalent pathogens including Staphylococcus aureus, Haemophilus influenzae, and Pseudomonas aeruginosa. Targeted antibiotic treatment and preventing exacerbations need an understanding of the microbiological profile of individuals with bronchiectasis.

A comprehensive method including clinical assessment, imaging investigations, pulmonary function testing, and microbiological testing is used to diagnose bronchiectasis. Imaging scans provide extensive anatomical information, and a comprehensive physical examination and a careful history of the patient set the foundation for subsequent investigations. Tests of pulmonary function measure the functional effect of bronchiectasis, whereas tests of microbiology pinpoint the microorganisms responsible for the condition so that customized treatments may be implemented. Through the combination of many diagnostic techniques, bronchiectasis may be fully understood, enabling patients with this chronic respiratory illness to receive individualized and successful care methods.

CHAPTER FIVE
INTERVENTION AND SUPERVISION

Chronic bronchiectasis is a respiratory disease marked by permanent bronchial dilatation, which impairs mucus clearance and increases the risk of infection and inflammation. A multidisciplinary strategy is used in the treatment and management of bronchiectasis, including medication, chest physical therapy, surgery, and lifestyle changes.

The therapy of bronchiectasis heavily relies on pharmacological interventions. Antibiotics, such as macrolides, are frequently administered to manage and avert bacterial infections, which are a frequent side effect of bronchiectasis. Because of their anti-inflammatory qualities, macrolides may help prevent exacerbations.

However, the possible negative consequences of its long-term usage must be carefully considered. Beta-agonists and anticholinergics are examples of bronchodilators, which work to reduce airflow blockage and enhance symptoms. Mucolytics are used to improve mucus clearance and lower the risk of infections and exacerbations.

Examples of these are hypertonic saline and recombinant human DNase. The goal of these pharmacological therapies is to enhance the quality of life for patients by addressing certain components of the disease associated with bronchiectasis.

A key component of the non-pharmacological care of bronchiectasis is chest physical therapy.

To help clear mucus from the airways, methods like vibration, percussion, and postural drainage are used. This lessens airway blockage and helps to avoid infection. Respiratory therapists frequently provide chest physical therapy, which is essential to the ongoing care of bronchiectasis.

In severe instances of bronchiectasis, particularly when conservative therapies are ineffective, surgical alternatives are taken into consideration. Lung resection, lobectomies, and, in the worst situations, lung transplants are examples of surgical procedures.

By removing diseased lung tissue, these operations seek to enhance both overall lung function and quality of life. Surgery is often saved for situations in which all other treatments have failed or in which the illness has progressed considerably.

Changing one's lifestyle is essential to controlling bronchiectasis. The goals of exercise and rehabilitation programs are to improve respiratory muscle strength and cardiovascular fitness. Frequent exercise can help to promote general well-being, lessen symptoms, and improve lung function.

An emphasis on keeping a well-balanced diet to promote immune function and general health is one of the most important nutritional issues.

To manage the energy needs associated with chronic respiratory diseases, an adequate diet is essential.

bronchiectasis therapy and management are complex and need an all-encompassing strategy that takes into account the disease's many facets. The goals of pharmacological therapies, such as bronchodilators, mucolytics, and antibiotics, are to improve mucus clearance, reduce symptoms, and control infections.

The promotion of airway clearing is greatly aided by chest physical therapy, with surgery being saved for more serious situations.

The management of bronchiectasis involves lifestyle adjustments that include exercise, rehabilitation, and dietary considerations.

The ultimate goal of these modifications is to enhance the general health and quality of life of those who are afflicted with this chronic respiratory ailment.

CHAPTER SIX
LIVING WITH BRONIACETASIS

Chronic bronchiectasis is a respiratory disease marked by permanent bronchial dilatation and destruction, which results in mucus buildup and heightened susceptibility to infections.

Those who are diagnosed with bronchiectasis encounter several difficulties in adequately controlling their disease. To assist patients in dealing with the psychological and physical challenges of having bronchiectasis, coping mechanisms are essential. Individuals with this disease typically use a variety of coping strategies to manage the symptoms and changes in lifestyle that come with it. These tactics may be having an optimistic outlook, creating a support system, and taking part in activities that improve general well-being.

Adaptive Techniques

People who have bronchiectasis must learn coping mechanisms to lessen the effects of their symptoms and enhance their quality of life. Developing an optimistic outlook is one crucial coping strategy. The chronic nature of bronchiectasis must be accepted by patients, who then need to concentrate on the areas of their lives that they can manage. This upbeat mindset can support improved mental health and a proactive attitude to handling the difficulties brought on by the illness. Patients can also gain a lot from attending support groups, where they can talk to others going through similar struggles, share experiences, and get emotional support.

Creating a solid support system is another essential coping technique. Support from friends, family, and medical experts is crucial for helping people with bronchiectasis manage their disease. Supportive relationships make patients feel connected, which improves their mental and emotional health.

They also offer practical aid, emotional support, and encouragement. Effective illness management also depends on having regular communication with healthcare providers.

This guarantees that treatment plans are continuously reviewed in light of the patient's changing requirements.

Participating in activities that enhance general well-being represents an additional coping mechanism for people with bronchiectasis. Improving immune system responses and respiratory performance can be achieved by leading a healthy lifestyle that includes frequent exercise, a balanced diet, and enough sleep. Patients and medical professionals should collaborate closely to create individualized exercise regimens that take into account each patient's unique physical capabilities and limits. Incorporating stress-reduction strategies, such as mindfulness and relaxation exercises, can also have a good effect on mental and physical health.

Assistive Healthcare

A comprehensive strategy is used in supportive treatment for bronchiectasis with the goals of reducing symptoms, averting complications, and enhancing general quality of life. The treatment of respiratory symptoms is a crucial component of supportive care. Medical professionals may recommend bronchodilators and mucolytic drugs to treat respiratory disorders and lessen mucus viscosity, which makes it easier for the airways to clear. Supportive care also benefits from pulmonary rehabilitation programs, which include information, emotional support, and planned exercise regimens to improve physical endurance and respiratory function.

To provide supportive care for patients with bronchiectasis, regular monitoring, and early intervention are crucial. Patients receive frequent laboratory evaluations, chest imaging, and pulmonary function testing to track the course of their disease and spot possible exacerbations. Healthcare professionals can minimize the influence on a patient's lung function and general well-being by rapidly adjusting treatment strategies upon timely diagnosis of infections or changes in symptoms. As a preventative approach, vaccination against respiratory infections—especially pneumonia and influenza—is essential to supportive treatment.

Having psychosocial support is essential to managing bronchiectasis holistically. It is crucial to take mental health into account because having a chronic respiratory disease can cause social isolation, anxiety, and sadness.

People can exchange coping mechanisms, talk about emotional difficulties, and get advice from mental health specialists in support groups and counseling programs. By including mental health assistance in the entire treatment plan, bronchiectasis's psychological effects may be addressed, and a more all-encompassing approach to wellbeing is encouraged.

Patient Empowerment And Education

A key component of managing bronchiectasis is patient education, which gives patients the capacity to take an active role in their care and choose their treatments with knowledge.

Patients need to be fully informed about their ailment, including its origins, symptoms, and possible implications, according to healthcare practitioners. With this information, individuals may effectively manage their condition on their own by identifying early indicators of exacerbations and seeking prompt medical attention.

Patients with bronchiectasis should receive education on a variety of topics, including how to clear the airways, how to use an inhaler correctly, and how important it is to take medicine as prescribed.

Patients must learn how to self-monitor, which includes keeping track of their symptoms and appreciating the value of routine examinations and diagnostic procedures. Moreover, educational programs have to prioritize lifestyle changes like quitting smoking and altering the surroundings to minimize exposure to respiratory irritants.

Building a sense of independence and self-efficacy in patients with bronchiectasis is essential to their empowerment in terms of health management. Healthcare professionals can assist patients in creating individualized action plans that specify what to do in the event of a change in health status or an aggravation of symptoms. When combined with continuous patient education, these action plans let patients take a more active role in their treatment, which improves the way their condition is managed.

managing bronchiectasis requires an all-encompassing strategy that includes patient education, supportive care, and coping mechanisms.

The amalgamation of these notions leads to a more comprehensive and patient-focused treatment paradigm, catering to the medical, psychological, and educational requirements of those suffering from bronchiectasis. People with bronchiectasis can work toward a higher quality of life and better long-term health outcomes by developing coping mechanisms, getting supportive treatment, and actively engaging in their education and empowerment.

CHAPTER SEVEN
RESEARCH AND FUTURE DIRECTIONS

A chronic respiratory disease called bronchiectasis is characterized by aberrant bronchial and bronchiole dilatation, which can result in lung function decrease and recurrent respiratory infections. Researching different facets of bronchiectasis is essential to improving our knowledge of the condition and creating novel treatment strategies as medical science advances. In this environment, the direction of bronchiectasis care is greatly influenced by current research trends, new treatments and technology, and optimism for the future.

Trends In Current Research

The main areas of interest for bronchiectasis research at the moment are new therapeutic approaches, biomarker identification for early diagnosis, and comprehension of the underlying processes. The complex interactions among microbial colonization, host immunological response, and structural lung damage in individuals with bronchiectasis are being studied by researchers. Thanks to developments in proteomics and genomics, tailored medication is now possible. Research is being done to find molecular and genetic markers linked to the onset and course of bronchiectasis. To further understand its involvement in the pathophysiology of the disease, there is an increasing focus on analyzing the microbiome of bronchiectasis patients.

Researchers are also devoting a great deal of study to the control of inflammatory pathways, and they are investigating the use of specific anti-inflammatory drugs to lessen lung damage and lower the frequency of exacerbations.

Clinical trials evaluating the effectiveness of current medications in managing bronchiectasis are in progress, providing insight into possible repurposing prospects.

Furthermore, research examining the effects of comorbidities, such as immunological dysregulation and gastric reflux, adds to a thorough comprehension of the complex nature of bronchiectasis.

New Technologies And Therapies

As new treatments and technology become available, the field of managing bronchiectasis is changing. Long-used in the treatment of cystic fibrosis, inhaled antibiotics are now being used to treat persistent bacterial infections in bronchiectasis patients. Researchers are looking into new antimicrobial compounds with a wider spectrum and improved bioavailability to deal with the problems caused by germs that are resistant to many drugs. The care of bronchiectasis still revolves around mucus clearance, and new developments in airway clearance devices, such as positive expiratory pressure devices and high-frequency chest wall oscillation, provide patients with more efficient alternatives.

The goal of immunomodulatory treatments, which are becoming more popular, is to adjust the immune system in cases of bronchiectasis. Monoclonal antibodies that target particular inflammatory pathways have the potential to improve lung function and decrease the frequency of exacerbations.

The potential of cellular treatments, such as mesenchymal stem cell transplantation, to encourage tissue repair and alter the inflammatory environment in the lungs is being investigated. Digital health and telehealth technologies are coming together to improve patient monitoring, encourage treatment plan adherence, and enable prompt interventions.

Optimism For The Future

There is optimism for a more promising future in the treatment of bronchiectasis because of the continuous research and new medicines.

Novel pharmacological targets will probably be found as a result of a greater comprehension of disease mechanisms, opening the door to more specialized and individualized treatment approaches. Precision medicine advances may make it possible to create treatments that are specific to each patient's profile, improving treatment results.

Patients with bronchiectasis may benefit from the study of regenerative medicine, which has the potential to restore damaged lung tissue.

Tissue engineering techniques and stem cell treatments have the potential to completely change the way that lung disease is treated while also providing a cure or considerable improvement in lung function.

Proactive management techniques may be made possible by the precision of early illness diagnosis and progression prediction made possible by the incorporation of artificial intelligence and machine learning into diagnostic and prognostic models.

To translate research discoveries into real-world therapeutic advantages, pharmaceutical firms, researchers, and physicians must work together. Encouraging patient participation and advocacy is also essential to guarantee that new treatments meet the requirements and preferences of bronchiectasis patients.

It is hoped that as research focuses on understanding the intricacies of this ailment, a thorough and potent treatment regimen will be developed, converting bronchiectasis from a debilitating, lifelong illness to one that is manageable or perhaps curable.

CONCLUSION

As a complex and multidimensional respiratory disease, bronchiectasis continues to require ongoing study to enhance diagnostic precision, elucidate pathogenic pathways, and provide efficacious treatment strategies.

Targeted therapies are becoming possible because of the increasing molecular knowledge of the illness that is being highlighted by current research developments.

New approaches to treating bronchiectasis and enhancing patient outcomes are provided by emerging medicines and technology, which range from cutting-edge medications to sophisticated airway-clearing equipment.

The possibility of transforming research discoveries into novel healthcare procedures is a source of optimism for the future.

There is hope that the treatment of bronchiectasis will change dramatically with an emphasis on precision medicine, regenerative medicines, and the use of cutting-edge technologies.

However, achieving this promise will need persistent interdisciplinary cooperation, proactive patient engagement, and a dedication to closing the knowledge gap between research and clinical practice.

The scientific community, medical experts, and patients are working together to uncover the complexity of bronchiectasis, and their combined efforts are providing hope for a better understanding and treatment of this difficult respiratory ailment in the future.